# The Paleo Athlete Meal Plan

## 28+ Quick & Easy, High Protein Meals For Building Muscle And Staying Lean!

Max Henrich

Copyright © 2014

*"**The Paleo Diet**, The World's Healthiest Diet - Is Based Upon Eating Wholesome, Contemporary Foods From The Food Groups That Our Hunter-Gatherer Ancestors Would Have Thrived On During The Paleolithic Era, Or Stone Age"*

-Dr. Loren Cordain Ph.D (founder of The Paleo Diet)

# Disclaimer

The contents outlined in this book are well-researched and the recommendations therein are founded on sound science and known ideas surrounding proper nutrition, detoxing and cleansing diets.

However, this book is not intended as a substitute for the medical advice of physicians, certified dieticians, and nutritionists who have spent a large portion of their professional careers studying proper nutrition, detox and cleansing. As a basic guide, this ebook is guaranteed to be more than sufficient for detox enthusiasts.

For more complex medical situations, the author recommends that readers should consult a physician, dietician or nutritionist in matters relating to his/her health and particularly with respect to any symptoms or conditions that may require special medical attention or specific diagnosis.

# Table of Contents

# What is the Paleo Diet?

You've probably heard of the Paleo diet more than a few times in the past, which is why you're now reading this awesome Paleo Diet cookbook for everyday athletes. So what is the Paleo diet all about and what can it do to help you perform better as an everyday athlete?

Dr. Loren Cordain, the founder of the Paleo diet, defines it as..

> *"The world's healthiest diet -it is based upon eating wholesome, contemporary foods from the food groups that our hunter-gatherer ancestors would have thrived on during the Paleolithic era, or Stone Age."*

The premise of the Paleo diet is very simple: since the latest research seems to indicate that our industrialized diets have coincided with the rise of many lifestyle-related diseases like Type II diabetes, obesity, and heart ailments, then reverting to our conventional diets long before the onset of industrialization and large-scale commercialization may help offset these diseases.

Dr. Cordain, in here decades-long research, actually specifically pointed out that the "caveman" of the Paleolithic period did not suffer from any of the following chronic diseases now common to Western civilization:

- Obesity

- Cardiovascular disease (heart disease, stroke, high blood pressure, congestive heart failure, atherosclerosis)

- Type II diabetes

- Cancer

- Autoimmune diseases (multiple sclerosis, rheumatoid arthritis, Crohn's disease, ulcerative colitis, etc.)

- Osteoporosis

- Acne

- Myopia (nearsightedness), macular degeneration, glaucoma

- Varicose veins, hemorrhoids, diverticulosis, gastric reflux

- Gout

# The Modern Paleo Diet

So, what does this mean for the modern version of the Paleo diet?

We'll, Dr. Cordain proposed that a diet based on wholesome, contemporary foods might just be the answer to reducing the risk and prevalence for these now-common chronic illnesses. These foods include fresh meats preferably of the grass-fed variety like beef, lamb or game meat, or the free-ranging variety like pork and poultry.

In addition, the Paleo diet also recommends eating healthy portions of fish, seafood, fresh fruits and vegetables, seeds and nuts, and healthy oils like olive oil, coconut oil, avocado oil, macadamia oil, walnut oil and flaxseed oil which would have been accessible to Paleolithic communities mainly from their diets.

Dairy products as well as cereal grains, legumes, refined sugars and processed foods were not part of our ancestral menu and hence are not included in the modern definition of the Paleo diet.

So in summary, the Paleo diet preaches a diet consisting of the following essential points and facets:

- **Higher protein intake.** Protein comprises 15 % of the calories in the average western diet, which is considerably lower than the average values of 19-35 % found in hunter-gatherer diets. Meat, seafood, and other animal products help augment our current protein intake in order to elevate it closer to the odern-day Paleo standard.

- **Lower carbohydrate intake and lower glycemic index.** Non-starchy fresh fruits and vegetables represent the bulk carbohydrate source of Paleo dieters and will provide about 35-45 % of our daily calorie needs. It is also important to note that almost all of these foods have low glycemic indices and will therefore NOT lead to spikes in your blood sugar levels.

- **Higher fiber intake.** Dietary fiber is one of the most important features of the Paleo diet just as it once was a major part of Paleolithic diets thousands of years ago. Naturally, these can't be found in the refined grains of today and even whole grains may have a problem matching the fiber intake of old Paleolithic diets mainly due to the sheer amount of genetic intervention that has occurred in the past decades. Non-starchy vegetables remain the golden standard as a primary dietary fiber source as these contain eight times more fiber than whole grains and 31 times more than refined grains. Even fruits contain twice as much fiber as whole grains and seven times more than refined grains.

- **Moderate to higher fat intake.** This rule comes with the caveat that majority of the fat intake should be in the form of monounsaturated and polyunsaturated fats with balanced Omega-3 and Omega-6 fats levels. Modern science has clearly shown that it isn't the total amount of fat in our diets that raises blood cholesterol levels and increases the risk for heart disease. Rather, it's the "type" of fat that's relevant to the increased risk for these illnesses. The Paleo diet recommends cutting back on trans-fats and Omega-6 polyunsaturated fats and instead increases the amount of healthy monounsaturated and Omega-3 fats. Recent studies have shown that saturated fats have little to zero adverse effects on cardiovascular disease which is why coconut oil is a part of the Paleo recommendation.

- **Higher potassium and lower sodium intake.** Increased salt in our diets is the primary culprit for elevated sodium intake. Conversely, fresh unprocessed foods naturally contain up to 10 times more potassium than sodium and this ratio is better for our bodies. Potassium is a vital part of the function of the heart, kidneys, and other organs and low potassium in the body has a strong correlation to illnesses like high blood pressure, heart disease, and stroke. Modern Western diets actually have about a 2:1 sodium-to-potassium ratio and the elevated sodium intake is a likely cause for many heart-related illnesses.

- **Net dietary alkaline load that balances dietary acid.** Many modern diets preach the importance of balance and dietary alkalinity and this should not come as a surprise. Acidic foods promote a variety of conditions such as bone and muscle loss, high blood pressure, and increased risk for kidney stones, and may also aggravate asthma due mainly to its inflammatory nature.

- **Higher consumption of vitamins, minerals and antioxidants.** – Whole grains are not a good substitute for grass-produced or free-ranging meats, fruits, and veggies because whole grains lack vitamin A, vitamin C, or vitamin B12. For a more balance vitamin and mineral profile in your diet, fresh fruits and vegetables and grass-produced meats are the best way to go.

So now that you've gotten a more detailed look at the Paleo diet, it's time to dig deeper and understand why the Paleo is the best diet for everyday athletes like you and me.

In the succeeding sections, we will talk more about the importance of protein for muscle building and specifically how one can build muscle while on the Paleo diet, the best nutrient profile for an athlete's diet, and the meal plan that's Paleo-compliant and suitable for an athlete in training.

# Paleo For The Everyday Athlete?

This book, seeks to help you take advantage of the Paleo diet as a way to become a better "everyday athlete." Whether you are into recreational sports or you compete in local sporting events to get to the podium or just beat a Personal Best, or you are trying out for the local team, or you have dreams to turn Pro.

Whatever your fitness goals may be - this Paleo Diet ebook will help you take the baby steps necessary to help you get from where you are today to where you want to be in the near future.

Here's what you can expect to find in this short but concise ebook on the Paleo diet for everyday athletes:

- A concise but informative discussion on the basis of the Paleo diet as explained by the Paleo found Dr. Loren Cordain.

- An informative guide on how the Paleo diet can help you build muscle and improve your performance as an athlete.

- A meal plan consisting of 30 great Paleo recipes that you can easily prepare on your own in the comforts of your own kitchen.

- Enough knowledge to equip you for long-term Paleo dieting. What you will learn from this ebook will go a long way towards shaping your strategy for transitioning to a healthier diet and lifestyle.

So, now that we got the basics out of the way, let's get started by answering the most important question that's been dogging you since you first read this ebook.

# Will Paleo Work For ALL Athletes?

In one simple word, *YES!*

Our Stone Age ancestors were natural athletes who had to exert tremendous amounts of effort and energy to get things done throughout the day. Nothing was handed to them. They can't just walk into a Stone-Age supermarket to buy all the stuff that they needed to survive; instead, they had to work for everything.

Hunting was a laborious task that often took days. Cavemen had to walk miles from their homes (or caves) to get to fertile grazing grounds of the prey that they wanted to hunt. There were no cars or trains to take them from Point A to Point B. All they had were their own two feet. In addition, they had to carry their own supplies to last them through the hunt and their hunting tools and equipment also weighed on their backs quite considerably.

Gatherers also didn't have it easy. Gathering whatever was edible at the forest floor wasn't a walk in the park since every single animal in the forest most likely competed for those resources. Gatherers actually had to climb trees to get fruits. They had to carry makeshift baskets to transport their cargo. They also walked some distance to get to the produce that they wanted.

Even tending to the fire most have likely required a lot of energy particularly in colder climes were getting the fire to burn continuously was a second-by-second challenge.

Our ancestors may not have competed in local marathons or swim meets but they were just as active, if not more active, and their bodies needed constant nourishment to allow them to get back up the next day and do it all over again.

And the proof that the Paleo diet worked for them is you, me, and us!

We are here today because our ancestors figured out a way that helped sustain their demanding and punishing lifestyles. If their diets failed, they would have easily starved out, their bodies growing frail with each passing day; and yet, we've always believed that our ancestors were strong and muscular and well-built because their diets allowed them to develop such strong bodies to cope up with the demanding tasks.

## SO... DOES THIS MEAN THE PALEO DIET WILL WORK FOR ME?

You can bet it does!

And you can add yourself to the list of many everyday success stories that gets poured in. These athletes adapted the Paleo lifestyle and relied on its unique diet properties to help them achieve their fitness goals, even as everyday athletes.

Let's learn more about the specifics - To do that, let's talk about nutrition as the main fuel that drives an athlete's inner core.

# Is High Protein Needed For Muscle Building?

Muscles are made up of protein molecules also known as amino acids. Just like vitamins and minerals, the body cannot make its own amino acids. Instead, it has to rely on amino acids consumed from food. When we eat protein, the body first has to break down the complex protein molecules into its component amino acids, and will then use those amino acids to make its own proteins including muscle tissues.

Of course, why athletes need to build muscle requires little explanation. All athletic abilities are founded on a few basic traits that boil down to the type of muscles that you have. Some of the more important traits include strength or power, speed, and endurance. The other traits like agility, dexterity, and even athleticism are all results of the primary traits that athletes need to have in order to perform well in their chosen sport.

So now that that's apparent, we go to the core question that constitutes the main purpose of this ebook.

# How To Build Muscle With The Paleo Diet?

The truth is that you cannot solely build muscle using the Paleo diet. You have to do it in combination with your workouts. It is the workout that primes the muscle for muscle-building, and it is the diet that provides the building blocks for the actual muscle building to occur. That "actual muscle building" phase actually happens post-workout during the recovery stage.

### *SO, HOW DOES THIS WORK?*

Well, workouts are intended to train your body to outperformance its previous best and develop a "new best." Every time you work out by running on the track or lifting weights at the gym, your body develops micro-tears in the muscle tissues. This is normal. As the body works hard to do what you are telling it to do, wear and tear inevitably comes in as a by-product.

But that's a good thing. Those tears now signal the rest of your body to send in the cavalry to repair, rebuild and recover the damage in preparation for the next workout. Having known that your muscles are supposed to do better next time so it can handle the load, your body will try to build bigger muscle tissues out of those tears. It will add new muscle strands and strengthen existing ones by bulking them up. For your body to do this during the recovery phase, you need to be properly nourished.

That's where the Paleo diet comes in.

# The Simple Stages Of Muscle Building Nutrition

Here's how a Paleo diet can help you build lean muscle mass as an athlete.

## STAGE I: PALEO PRE-WORKOUT NUTRITION

In brief, the low to moderate glycemic index carbohydrates that feature heavily in the Paleo diet works well with conventional practices on pre-workout nutrition. This helps give your body just enough calories to power your workouts later in the day.

As a suggestion, take in about 200 to 300 calories of low-fiber food for every hour of workout that you plan to do. Make sure to eat 2 to 3 hours before your workout, but if eating prior is not possible, then take in about 200 calories 10 minutes before the workout or race begins.

## STAGE II: DURING-WORKOUT PALEO NUTRITION

Water is the only thing that you need during short to medium-duration workouts. The moment you take your workouts longer than a couple of hours, you will need to also take in some potassium sources such as those that can be found in banana.

You will also tremendously benefit from maintaining your access to medium-GI foods so you can keep your blood sugar level up while working out.

## STAGE III: POST WORKOUT PALEO NUTRITION

In the first 30 minutes post-workout, you can plan for a good meal that combines hydration, carbohydrates and lean protein sources in one. Post workout is critical because it dictates how well you will recover afterward.

A great Paleo meal 30-minute after the workout will help ensure that your body is properly fueled for the long recovery period that it has to endure in repairing muscle damage and building new ones.

## STAGE IV: EXTENDED RECOVERY PALEO NUTRITION

For the succeeding hours after your workout, continue to focus your diet on carbohydrates, especially moderate to high glycemic load carbohydrates along with protein at a 4-5:1 carb-protein ratio.

This works if, say, you had your workout in the afternoon and now need to eat a great dinner to continue piling in the nourishment.

## STAGE V: LONG-TERM PALEO NUTRITION

Recovery for the remainder of your day, or until your next Stage I, consists of conventional Paleo Diet with the recipes outlined in the succeeding section. Just by sticking to the Paleo routine, you are already giving your body all the nourishment that it needs to build muscles and help improve your performance for the next workouts.

# The Macronutrient Ratio For Athletes

Macronutrient ratios are never the same for any one person due to varying factors that influence how these nutrients are utilized. Same as the metabolism of an athlete versus the average Joe is completely different. Still, there are acceptable ranges that you can consider as a rough guide when it comes to your Paleo diet.

Macronutrients are:

1. **Carbohydrates**
2. **Proteins**
3. **Fats**

Here are some of the guidelines that you should keep in mind when developing your unique mean plan.

# Carbohydrates

Most of the calories in your diet should come from carbohydrates. The expected range for carbohydrates is about 45% to 65% of your daily calorie intake. Take note that carbohydrates provide 4 calories per 1 g, so if you require 2,000 calories per day, your carbohydrate intake should be in the range of 225 g at the 45% level to 325 g of carbs at the 65% level.

In addition, the Food and Nutrition Board recommends a carb-to-fiber ratio that is optimal. For every 1,000 calories you eat, you should consume 14 g of fiber. For the same example of 2,000 calories per day, you should consume 28 g of fiber.

## Proteins

The Paleo diet doesn't make any love for protein a secret. It recommends eating more lean meat that corresponds to about 10% to 35% of your daily calorie intake.

Like carbs, protein provides about 4 calories per 1 g so if you consume 2,000 calories per day; protein intake should fall between 50 g and 175 g.

## Fats

Believe it or not, fat has the second highest recommended dietary range in an athlete's your diet. Your fat consumption should be about 20% to 35% of your daily calorie intake. Healthy fats are the most energy-dense macronutrient making it highly favorable for fueling workouts. A gram of fat provides about 9 calories so if you consume 2,000 calories per day, your fat intake should range from 44 g at the 20% level and to 78 g at the 35% level.

The Paleo diet covers all the necessary fat types that you need to take in more and the fat types that you should watch out and avoid. As a rule, saturated fat should comprise less than 10% of your daily calories while trans-fat should contribute less than 1% of calories. If you consume 2,000 calories per day, you should consume less than 22 g of saturated fat and less than 2 g of trans-fat.

Now that you know these, it's time to look at some recipes that can help you become a better athlete just by being able to eat in a way that complements your workout-heavy lifestyle.

# 30 Paleo Recipes Designed for Muscle-Building

Here are 30 awesome Paleo recipes that you can use to help you become a better athlete. We've broken them down into three sections, each for breakfast, lunch and dinner. All the meals outlined in this book contained approximately ~30 grams of protein per meal.

This is important to mention because this nutrient is vital to building lean muscle mass. So without further ado, let's start studying the tasty meals ahead. I suggest you play around and try them all so you can get a better feel for what suits your unique taste.

# Breakfast Paleo Recipes

The following Paleo recipes are perfect for a morning fixer-upper and are ideal if you want properly fuel your body for the rest of the day.

# Baked Eggs and Prosciutto

This is a recipe loaded with plenty of proteins to help you build muscles. The egg and prosciutto are great complementary ingredients. Make sure to get the unsalted prosciutto to limit your intake of sodium from the table salt.

**Yield:** 1 serving

**Ingredients:**

2 slices prosciutto

1 egg (organic eggs from pasture-raised chickens)

½ cup lean ground beef

chives, chopped

black pepper, freshly ground

1 tsp. heavy cream

**Directions:**

1. Pre-heat your oven to 370-degrees F.
2. Line a ramekin with two slices of prosciutto. It doesn't need to be overly elegant; drapes along the side are just fine.

3. Crack an egg into the ramekin and add a teaspoon of your preferred cream. Heavy cream is the preferred ingredient here.

4. Flavor with pepper, lean ground beef and chopped chives and pop the ramekin into the oven for about 15 minutes. Once cooked, take out the ramekin and allow standing for about 5 minutes before serving.

**Nutrition Facts:** Total calories 145, protein 36 g, carbs 12g, fat 3g, saturated fat 0.5 g, fiber 2g, salt 0.2 g.

# Paleo Breakfast Hash

Looking for a way to cook together a variety of your favorite Paleo ingredients? This hash recipe is perfect for mixing and combining multiple ingredients together so you get a protein-packed dish in the most important meal of the day. Enjoy!

**Yield:** 1 serving

**Ingredients:**

1 large sweet potato, chopped

½ cup peppers, chopped

½ cup onions, chopped

1 large handful fresh organic spinach

1 tomato, finely chopped

1 ½ tsp. extra-virgin olive oil

2 garlic cloves, crushed

2 organic chicken sausages, chopped

Himalayan sea salt

pepper, freshly ground

1 organic egg, cooked easy

## Directions:

1. Sauté the garlic in olive oil over medium heat for about a minute before adding the chopped sweet potato. After another 5 minutes, add the peppers, tomato, and onions and continue sautéing for another 5 minutes.

2. Toss in the organic chicken sausages. Take note you also have the option to use other types of meat here such as unsalted bacon. Depending on the type of meat that you use, cooking time should be between 5 to 7 minutes.

3. Add the fresh spinach and continue sautéing for another 2 minutes. Flavor with salt and pepper.

4. Take the pan out of the heat and allow cooling before serving over organic easy cooked eggs.

**Nutrition Facts:** Total calories 195, protein 45g, carbs 24g, fat 6g, saturated fat 0.8 g, fiber 4g, salt 2 g.

# Paleo Omelet

Everyone has their own omelet recipe so this one should be fairly easy. For best results, just mix in a few other ingredients to elevate the macronutrient profile of your breakfast to give it a more "complete feel."

**Yield:** 1 serving

**Ingredients:**

4 omega-3 eggs

1 tbsp. extra virgin olive oil

1 cup spinach leaves, chopped

½ cup boiled chicken breast, cut into pieces

1 tsp. fresh basil, finely chopped

1 small avocado

black pepper, freshly ground

**Directions:**

1. In a mixing bowl, whisk the eggs until they form a light foamy froth.
2. Using a skillet over medium heat, use the olive oil to cook the eggs and form an omelet. When

the eggs have set, add the spinach and chicken breast on the side and flavor with pepper and basil. Cook for about 1 minute and then transfer on to the omelet before folding.

3. Serve with avocado.

**Nutrition Facts:** Total calories 168, protein 34g, carbs 22g, fat 7g, saturated fat 2 g, fiber 5g, salt 1 g

# Protein-Rich Paleo Pumpkin Pancakes

Cavemen may not have had the pleasure of eating pancakes back in the day but they sure had access to all the ingredients outlined here. And with all the goodness in a great stack of pancakes, who's to say you can't bank on these to give you all the protein you need to fuel your workouts?

**Yield:** 2 servings

**Ingredients:**

   4 strips bacon

   ¼ cup coconut flour

   3 eggs

   ½ tsp. cinnamon

   ¼ tsp. Himalayan salt

   ¼ cup pumpkin puree

   ½ tsp. apple cider vinegar

   1 tbsp. coconut oil, melted

   ¼ tsp. pumpkin pie spice

   ¼ cup almond milk

¼ cup pure maple syrup

**Directions:**

1.  Whisk together the dry ingredients including the coconut flour, Himalayan salt, cinnamon and nutmeg. In a separate bowl, also whisk together the wet ingredients including the eggs, coconut oil, apple cider vinegar, maple syrup and pumpkin puree.

2.  Add the dry mix and wet mix and mix well until smooth.

3.  Using a skillet over medium heat, with coconut oil, spoon the batter into the pan in your preferred pancake size. Just remember that denser and bigger pancakes take more time to cook than smaller thinner ones. Upon spooning, make sure to flatten and shape the batter to about 1/3 inch to facilitate even cooking. Once done, flip over to the other side.

4.  Serve with pure maple syrup and fried bacon on the side. Enjoy.

**Nutrition Facts:** Total calories 125, protein 30 g, carbs 15 g, fat 5g, saturated fat 2 g, fiber 2g, salt 1 g.

# Paleo Breakfast Casserole

This is a classic Paleo dish combining meat and vegetables and adding a modern culinary flair by whipping it all up into a nice casserole bundle. If you want a protein-rich and satisfying recipe to get you up to speed in the morning, this is the recipe for you.

**Yield:** 8 servings

**Ingredients:**

  1 pound breakfast sausage

  2 medium sweet potatoes, diced

  2 cups fresh baby spinach, chopped

  1 green onion, diced

  10 large eggs

  sea salt

  pepper, freshly ground

**Directions:**

  1.  Preheat your oven to 375 degrees (F) and grease a glass baking dish with coconut oil then set aside for a few minutes.

2. Meanwhile, start preparing the veggies. Dice the sweet potatoes, chop the spinach, and dice up green onion then set aside separately.

3. Using a skillet over medium heat, remove the sausage from the casing and add into the skillet. Cook until the sausage gains a brown color and then remove while still keeping the sausage grease on the skillet. Now, add the sweet potatoes and cook for about 10 minutes until tender.

4. Remove sweet potatoes and place them in a bowl. Mix the sweet potatoes with the spinach, chopped sausage, green onion, and flavored with salt and pepper to taste. Lay down the mixture into the glass dish, spreading evenly across the bottom to ensure even cooking throughout.

5. In another large bowl, whisk the eggs and then pour the resulting mixture evenly over the sausage and veggie layer. Bake in preheated oven for about 25 minutes.

6. Allow the mixture to cool slightly before serving. Cut into squares and serve.

**Nutrition Facts:** Total calories 192, <u>protein 53 g,</u> carbs 24 g, fat 9 g,  saturated fat 3 g, fiber 4 g, salt 2 g.

# Apple-Carrot-Banana Bread

Everyone needs a great go-to bread recipe, even when you are on the Paleo diet. And with the stern emphasis on staying away from refined and whole grains, you are not left with many chances for baking success. Well, not until now; enter apples, carrots and banana for an awesome loaf of bread that is a great compliment to all your breakfast dishes.

**Yield:** 8 servings

**Ingredients:**

2 small carrots, shredded

1 apple, shredded

1 ripe banana, mashed

4 medjool dates, pitted

5 eggs

½ cup coconut oil, melted

1 tsp. vanilla extract

½ cup walnuts

2 tbsp. maple syrup

½ cup coconut flour

¼ tsp. baking soda

¼ tsp. sea salt

1 tsp. cinnamon, ground

½ tsp. ginger, ground

¼ tsp. cloves, ground

**Directions:**

1. Preheat your oven to 350 degrees (F). Meanwhile, grease a bread loaf pan with coconut oil.

2. Prepare the veggies by shredding the carrots and apple and set aside.

3. In a food processor, add the banana, eggs, dates, the remaining coconut oil, vanilla extract, and maple syrup and process until dates are completely broken up and no large chunks are in mixture. Continue adding the coconut flour, baking soda, sea salt, cinnamon, walnuts, ginger, and cloves to the food processor and process until a batter forms. Remove blade from bowl and stir in shredded carrots and apple to complete the dough.

4. Pour the batter into the greased loaf pan and bake for about 45 minutes. You can sprinkle

additional cinnamon on top of loaf if you desire as well. Afterwards, allow the loaf to cool for about 15 minutes before cutting into the bread.

**Nutrition Facts:** Total calories 134, protein 31 g, carbs 29 g, fat 8 g, saturated fat 3 g, fiber 8 g, salt 1 g.

# Poached Egg with Peach and Prosciutto Salsa

This is an easy-to-make breakfast recipe if you are on the go but would want to make sure you are adequately fueled for the day ahead.

**Yield:** 1 serving

**Ingredients:**

For the poached egg:

> 2 medium-sized omega 3-enriched eggs
>
> 2 tbsp. flaxseed oil

For the peach and prosciutto salsa:

> 1 cup peaches, peeled, finely chopped
>
> ¼ cup red onions, chopped
>
> ¼ yellow or green peppers, chopped
>
> 4 slices prosciutto
>
> 1 tbsp. lime juice
>
> 2 tsp. fresh cilantro
>
> cayenne pepper

**Directions:**

1. For the poached egg: Bring half-an-inch of water in a pan to a boil. Rub a little flaxseed oil in the egg wells of an egg poacher, then crack the eggs into the egg wells and reduce heat to a slow boil. Place the poacher in the saucepan and cover. Medium-sized eggs should take about 6 minutes to poach.

2. Remove the egg poacher from the pan and take out the eggs with a flexible rubber spatula. Gently transfer the eggs to a plate and smother with peach salsa.

3. For the peach and prosciutto salsa: Toss all the salsa ingredients in a bowl and stir until all the ingredients are properly mixed. Chill for at least 6 hours before serving.

4. This is best enjoyed with a whey protein drink that you can quickly prepare by dissolving 2 tablespoons of whey powder into a glass of cold water.

**Nutrition Facts:** Total calories 153, protein 31 g, carbs 17 g, fat 4 g, saturated fat 1 g, fiber 1 g, salt 0 g.

# Gazpacho (Soup)

If you want an easy-to-make soup for breakfast, this is the dish for you. This recipe works really well when served with bread, preferably the apple-carrot-banana loaf which we also described in this section.

**Yield:** 2 servings

**Ingredients:**

4 large tomatoes, chopped

1 small onion, coarsely chopped

1 clove garlic, peeled

1 cup tomato juice, unsalted

2 tbsp. lemon juice

3 strips of bacon

1/2 cup egg whites

2 tbsp. olive oil

pepper

cayenne pepper to taste

1 sprig fresh parsley

4 ice cubes

1 medium cucumber, peeled and coarsely chopped

## Directions:

1. Blend all ingredients in a blender or food processor until vegetables are small but not pureed.
2. In a sauce pan, add the oil and sauté the bacon until crispy. Crumble.
3. To serve, sprinkle the crumbled bacon over the gazpacho.

**Nutrition Facts:** Total calories 134, protein 32 g, carbs 19 g, fat 3 g,  saturated fat 0.7 g, fiber 6 g, salt 0.3 g.

# Banana Paleo Shake

If you're the type that can go through your morning with just a power shake to fuel your body, this is the recipe for you. With all the ingredients together, this shake provides a great blend of protein, potassium, and calories designed to keep you awake and fired up for the brand new day ahead of you.

**Yield:** 1 serving

**Ingredients:**

2 large bananas, sliced

½ cup ice cubes

½ cup strong coffee

2 tbsp. cocoa powder

1-2 scoop whey protein powder

1 tbsp. honey

1 tbsp. coconut butter

**Directions:**

1. Make sure the coffee is at room temperature before making this shake. Another option is to

freeze the coffee into ice cubes and then using those to blend the ingredients together.

2. To prepare the shake, place all ingredients in a blender and process until smooth.

**Nutrition Facts:** Total calories 95, protein 36 g, carbs 19 g, fat 5 g, saturated fat 2 g, fiber 1 g, salt 0 g.

# Paleo Porridge

This Paleo porridge is a great alternative to shakes and smoothies. If you want something light but filling and full of all the nutrients you need to power your workouts, you can never go wrong with this Paleo porridge.

**Yield:** 1 serving

**Ingredients:**

2 slices prosciutto

½ cup egg whites

2 ripe bananas, mashed

2 cups coconut milk

¾ cup almond meal

¼ cup flax meal

1 tsp. cinnamon

½ tsp. ginger, grated

1/8 tsp. cloves, ground

1/8 tsp. nutmeg, ground

1/8 tsp. Celtic sea salt

1 tbsp. raw honey

assorted toppings (berries, unsweetened coconut flakes, nuts, seeds, etc.)

## Directions:

1. Combine all the ingredients in a medium saucepan and set the heat to low until the mixture simmers. Stir frequently.
2. The porridge is ready when the mixture has turned thick and bubbly.
3. Serve with the toppings and thin slices of prosciutto on top.

**Nutrition Facts:** Total calories 112, <u>protein 30 g,</u> carbs 26 g, fat 9 g, saturated fat 4 g, fiber 3 g, salt 0.5 g.

# Lunch Paleo Recipes

These recipes are perfect to tide you over from morning to afternoon. Depending on when you do your workouts, you'll need a fresh boost of energy to get you through the afternoon hours, which helps explain why these recipes are designed to be refreshing, filling, but also light to the stomach.

Remember, the main intention isn't to fill your stomach; rather, it's to complement give you enough energy to get you going prior to the all-important afternoon workout.

# African-Style Paleo Curry

This African-style curry is the perfect way to enjoy international flavors while you're at the office during lunchtime. With this recipe, there's no need to stray too far away from your diet by heading to the nearest restaurant for a great meal. Just simple prepare this early in the morning, pack it up, and pop it in the microwave for a sumptuous lunch that you can enjoy with great gusto.

**Yield:** 4 servings

**Ingredients:**

1 tbsp. olive oil

1 onion, chopped

2 cloves garlic, peeled, chopped

1 bay leaf

4 large tomatoes, peeled

2 tsp. curry powder

1/8 tsp. salt

2-pounds chicken breast, de-boned, skinless, cut

2 cups unsweetened coconut milk

1 lemon, juiced

**Directions:**

1. Heat the olive oil in a skillet over medium heat and sauté the onions, garlic, and bay leaf for about 2 minutes. Add in the tomatoes, curry powder, and salt and continue cooking for about 5 minutes. Toss the chicken and cook for 20 minutes until the chicken is no longer pink and juices run clear.

2. Reduce the heat to low and stir constantly. Blend the coconut milk slowly over a period of about 10 minutes.

3. Squeeze lemon or pour the lemon just before serving.

**Nutrition Facts:** Total calories 188, protein 46 g, carbs 31 g, fat 11 g, saturated fat 2 g, fiber 4 g, salt 0.3 g.

# Salmon and Capers Salad

Salads are great Paleo lunch recipes because they are easy to prepare and can be packed quickly for a meal on-the-run. This recipe uses salmon as your primary protein source so you can continue to get your protein requirements even while you're at the office and busy with work.

**Yield:** 3 servings

**Ingredients:**

   1 pound salmon fillet

   salt and pepper

   ½ lemon, juice, zest grated

   2 tbsp. capers, drained, rinsed

   1 celery stalk, chopped

   1 tsp. fresh dill, chopped

   2 tbsp. extra-virgin olive oil

**Directions:**

1. Season the salmon with salt and pepper and bake in a 350-degree (F) oven for about 8 minutes until opaque and flaky.
2. Once cooked, transfer into a bowl and mix all the remaining ingredients.
3. The dish can be served hot or cold depending on your preference.

**Nutrition Facts:** Total calories 147, protein 37 g, carbs 17 g, fat 7 g, saturated fat 0.5 g, fiber 3 g, salt 0.1 g.

# Chicken Salad

If you want chicken instead of salmon, here's a very simple equivalent recipe that you can try for lunch.

**Yield:** 3 servings

**Ingredients:**

2 cooked chicken breasts, chopped

2 celery stalks, chopped

½ cup pecans, chopped

½ cup dried cranberries

1/3 cup homemade mayonnaise

1 tsp. poppy seeds

1 tbsp. apple cider vinegar

1 tbsp. honey

**Directions:**

1. Combine all the ingredients together in a bowl. Enjoy!

**Nutrition Facts:** Total calories 153, <u>protein 39 g,</u> carbs 24 g, fat 10 g, saturated fat 3 g, fiber 5 g, salt 0.1 g.

# The Ultimate Paleo Meatloaf

You can prepare this meatloaf beforehand and pack it for lunch the next day. You can also pair it with any of the Paleo-approved bread recipes we mentioned in this ebook.

**Yield:** 8 servings

**Ingredients:**

1 ½ pounds ground beef

1 tbsp. Worcestershire sauce

½ cup tomato sauce

1/3 cup crushed pork skins, fried

2 eggs

2 ½ tbsp. chili powder

1 tbsp. garlic salt

1 tbsp. garlic pepper seasoning

**Directions:**

1. Preheat you oven to 375 degrees F. Meanwhile, mix together the ground beef, Worcestershire sauce, tomato sauce, crushed pork skins, and eggs in a large bowl and season with chili

powder, garlic salt, and garlic pepper. Mix thoroughly. Form into a loaf, and place into a greased loaf pan.

2. Bake for up to 40 minutes. When done, allow to stand for at least 5 minutes to cool down before slicing and serving.

**Nutrition Facts:** Total calories 202, <u>protein 48 g,</u> carbs 38 g, fat 9 g, saturated fat 4 g, fiber 3 g, salt 0.7 g.

# Baked Salmon

What can be simpler than baking salmon? You can reheat the dish in the office and enjoy a protein-packed dish to help fuel your workouts.

**Yield:** 3 servings

**Ingredients:**

> 2 cloves garlic, minced
>
> 6 tbsp. light olive oil
>
> 1 tsp. dried basil
>
> 1 tsp. salt
>
> 1 tsp. black pepper, ground
>
> 1 tbsp. lemon juice
>
> 1 tbsp. fresh parsley, chopped
>
> 2 fillets salmon

**Directions:**

1. In a bowl, prepare the marinade by mixing garlic, olive oil, basil, salt, pepper, lemon juice and parsley. Place the salmon fillets in a baking dish, and cover with the marinade. Marinate in the refrigerator for about 1 hour.

2. Preheat your oven to 375 degrees F.

3. Place the fillets in an aluminum foil and cover with marinade. Seal, and place into a glass dish, then bake for about 35 minutes.

**Nutrition Facts:** Total calories 175, <u>protein 52 g,</u> carbs 25 g, fat 5 g,  saturated fat 0.5 g, fiber 3 g, salt 1 g.

## Meat-Lover's Chili

Who doesn't love a good chili dish? And much more so when it is Paleo-approved and packed with protein for a sumptuous lunch! Enjoy this classic chili recipe that you can prepare the night before and heat up for a great meal wherever you may be mid-day of the following day.

**Yield:** 8 servings

**Ingredients:**

  2 large Italian sausages, chopped

  1 pound round steak, chopped

  2 pounds sirloin, ground

  2 cups yellow onion, chopped

  1 ½ cups bell pepper

  8 cloves garlic, minced

  2 cups tomatoes, chopped

  2 tbsp. chili powder

  1 tbsp. ancho chili pepper

  1 tbsp. cumin

  3 tsp. tomato paste

1 tsp. dried oregano

½ tsp. pepper, freshly ground

½ tsp. salt

2 bay leaves

## Directions:

1. Heat a pan over medium heat and add all the meat, onions, bell pepper, and garlic to pan. Cook until the meats are browned and crumbling. This should take about 25 to 30 minutes.

2. Add the chili powder, ancho chili pepper, cumin and tomato paste, oregano, salt, pepper and bay leaves and cook for 1 minute, stirring constantly. Add the tomatoes and bring to a boil. Afterwards, transfer the mixture to a crock pot or slow cooker and let cook for 6 hours on low.

3. Discard the bay leaves before serving.

**Nutrition Facts:** Total calories 215, protein 42 g, carbs 29 g, fat 12 g, saturated fat 4 g, fiber 6 g, salt 0.2 g.

# Herb, Garlic and Bacon Loin

This is the ultimate meat-lovers recipe and it's perfect for a protein-overload for the everyday athlete. Enjoy!

**Yield:** 10 servings

**Ingredients:**

  5-pound pork loin roast

  1 tbsp. olive oil

  1-pound sliced bacon

  3 cups chicken stock

  1 tbsp. dried rosemary

  1 tbsp. dried thyme

  6 fresh basil leaves

  6 fresh sage leaves

  4 cloves garlic, chopped

  8 fresh pearl onions, peeled

**Directions:**

1. Preheat your oven to 300 degrees F. Meanwhile, rub the pork loin with olive oil and place in a roasting pan. Then, drape slices of bacon over the top and pour in the combination of chicken stock, rosemary, thyme, basil, sage and garlic. Place onions around the sides and cover with lid or aluminum foil before putting into the oven.

2. Bake for about 90 minutes, then remove the lid or foil and continue baking for another 30 minutes until the bacon is browned.

3. For best results, prepare this recipe the night before so you can pack and re-heat it for lunch.

**Nutrition Facts:** Total calories 205, protein 53 g, carbs 36 g, fat 12 g, saturated fat 5 g, fiber 4 g, salt 0.2 g.

# Shrimp and Spinach Salad

Shrimp is a great source of protein if you want a simple alternative to everyday meat lunch recipes. Try this quick shrimp and spinach salad for a light lunch with all the protein goodness you can ever need.

**Yield:** 3 servings

**Ingredients:**

> 1-pound shrimp
>
> 1 bell pepper, diced
>
> ½ yellow onion, diced
>
> 4 big handfuls baby spinach leaves
>
> 2 tbsp. coconut oil
>
> 2 tbsp. coconut milk
>
> ½ tbsp. curry powder
>
> sea salt
>
> black pepper

**Directions:**

1. In a skillet, heat the coconut oil over medium heat and sauté the onions and bell peppers. Add the shrimp and the spinach and cook for about 3 minutes or until the shrimp curls up and gains a reddish pinkish color.
2. Add the coconut milk and spices. Mix well and serve!

**Nutrition Facts:** Total calories 144, <u>protein 31 g,</u> carbs 17 g, fat 9 g,  saturated fat 3 g, fiber 8 g, salt 0.6 g.

# Paleo-Approved Jambalaya

The Jambalaya is fast-gaining attention as a great protein source that's easy to prepare and great to the taste. This Paleo-approved version is great if you want strong and exotic flavors on your palate for lunch.

**Yield:** 4 servings

**Ingredients:**

   2 tsp. olive oil

   2 tsp. butter

   5/8 large onion, diced

   1 ¼ ouille sausage, cut

   4 cloves garlic, finely chopped

   2 cups tomatoes, crushed

   2 green bell peppers, seeded, diced

   1 zucchini, diced

   1 tbsp. plus 1 tsp. Cajun seasoning

   ¾ tsp. hot sauce

   2/3 cup chicken broth

   2 cups chicken breast, boiled, cooled, and chopped

2 cups shrimp, deveined, peeled, boiled, cooked

**Directions:**

1. Heat the olive oil and butter in a large saucepan over medium heat and sauté the onion and andouille sausage until brown. This should take about 10 minutes. Add the garlic and cook for another 2 minutes.

2. Into the pan, mix in the crushed tomatoes, green bell peppers, zucchinis, Cajun seasoning, hot sauce, and chicken broth and bring the mixture to a boil. Once boiling, reduce to a simmer and cook uncovered to reduce the liquid. This will take about 15 minutes.

3. Stir in chicken and shrimp and simmer for another 2 minutes.

4. Serve hot or chill and reheat later.

**Nutrition Facts:** Total calories 192, <u>protein 40 g,</u> carbs 33 g, fat 10 g, saturated fat 4 g, fiber 5 g, salt 0.5 g.

# Tuna Steaks

Tuna steaks are great alternatives to classic steaks. This simple recipe cooks in just 15 minutes so you can prepare this early in the morning and pack it to work or you can prepare it fresh if you are just staying at home for lunch. This specific recipe is designed for 4 servings but can easily be adjusted by varying the amount of tuna that you cook.

**Yield:** 4 servings

**Ingredients:**

　　3 tbsp. olive oil

　　2 cloves garlic, peeled, minced

　　2 tbsp. tarragon vinegar

　　½ tsp. dried tarragon

　　black pepper, freshly ground

　　1 ½ pound fresh tuna steaks

**Directions:**

1. In a bowl, mix together the olive oil, garlic, tarragon vinegar, dried tarragon and pepper. Soak the tuna steaks into the mixture and marinate for at least 4 hours.

2. Preheat an outdoor grill for high heat and lightly the oil grate. Grill the tuna steaks for about 8 minutes on each side until the tuna flakes easily and is opaque in the center.

3. Serve hot or pack for lunch.

**Nutrition Facts:** Total calories 125, protein 35 g, carbs 16 g, fat 5 g, saturated fat 0 g, fiber 1 g, salt 0 g.

# Dinner Paleo Recipes

Most everyday athletes do their work outs in the evening right before dinner so Paleo dinner recipes should be geared towards refueling for recovery purposes.

In addition, it is also important to keep the recipes simple so preparing your meals doesn't take a lot of your time after a tough day at the gym or on the field. We've kept those things in mind when we developed these dinner Paleo recipes for you.

# Kale Salad with Chicken

Here's a simple kale salad and chicken recipe designed to give you both protein and fiber in one fix. This recipe is also easy to prepare so if you just came from a long day, you know it doesn't take much time to get dinner on the table.

**Yield:** 2 servings

**Ingredients:**

6 cups kale, chopped

2 tbsp. extra-virgin olive oil

1 small lemon, juiced

1/8 tsp. sea salt (optional)

¼ tsp. black pepper, freshly ground

2 pcs. chicken breasts, boneless, skinless, cooked, sliced

¼ cup sunflower seeds, toasted

**Directions:**

1. Wash the kale and remove the woody stems, then chopped finely.

2. In a bowl, combine the kale with olive oil, lemon juice, sea salt (optional) and freshly ground black pepper. Toss to coat leaves completely. Then, divide the kale into two bowls and top each salad with a cooked chicken breast and sunflower seeds to serve.

**Nutrition Facts:** Total calories 163, protein 35 g, carbs 24 g, fat 8 g,  saturated fat 0 g, fiber 8 g, salt 0.4 g.

# Sardine Salad

Sardines and salad, now that's a refreshing recipe that you can rely on for protein after a tough workout; in addition, this one is so easy to prepare, you know you can immediately eat without having to spend a long time in the kitchen! Enjoy!

**Yield:** 2 servings

**Ingredients:**

3 medium tomatoes, diced

1 medium yellow squash, diced

1 large celery stalk, diced

1 head romaine lettuce, chopped,

¼ cup raw sauerkraut

1 cup cabbage, shredded

2 small avocados, diced

1 cup sardines in oil, chopped

1 tbsp. balsamic vinegar

½ lime, juiced

1 tsp. Dijon mustard

¼ tsp. sea salt (optional)

**Directions:**

1. Add all ingredients to a mixing bowl and toss to mix. Add salt if desired.
2. Divide into two bowls to serve.

**Nutrition Facts:** Total calories 134, protein 33 g, carbs 28 g, fat 9 g,  saturated fat 3 g, fiber 6 g, salt 0.4 g.

# Halibut with Dijon and Almonds

If you're a fan of fish, this recipe will make it so much simpler to prepare your dinner while still allowing you to enjoy a good fish dinner. To vary the Serving, simply choose a bigger or smaller fish.

**Yield:** 2 servings

**Ingredients:**

4 tbsp. olive oil

1-pound halibut (other types of white fish are also okay)

2 tbsp. Dijon mustard

2 tbsp. almonds, chopped

**Directions:**

1. Preheat you oven to 350° F. Meanwhile, lightly grease a baking sheet with olive or coconut oil. Lay the fish in the pan skin side down and spread the Dijon mustard over fish and sprinkle with almonds.

2. Bake the fish for about 15 minutes until flaky.

3. Serve hot.

**Nutrition Facts:** Total calories 161, <u>protein 38 g,</u> carbs 15 g, fat 5 g,  saturated fat 0 g, fiber 2 g, salt 0 g.

# Asian Stir-Fry

Here's a Paleo-approved Asian-style recipe for your palate. Enjoy!

**Yield:** 4 servings

**Ingredients:**

1-pound chicken breast, boneless, skinless

2 tbsp. coconut oil

1 medium onion, finely chopped

2 heads broccoli, sliced

2 medium carrots, sliced

2 heads baby bok choy, sliced

1 small zucchini, sliced

½ cup shiitake mushrooms, stemmed, thinly sliced

½ tsp. Celtic sea salt

1 ½ cups water

2 tbsp. arrowroot powder

2 tbsp. sesame oil, toasted

2 tbsp. ume plum vinegar

1 tbsp. honey

## Directions:

1. Rinse the chicken and pat dry then cut into 1-inch cubes and transfer to a plate.

2. On a skillet over medium heat, add coconut oil and sauté the onion for about 8 minutes to caramelize. Add the broccoli, carrots, and chicken and continue sautéing for another 10 minutes until almost tender. Continue adding the bok choy, mushrooms, zucchini, and salt and sauté for another 5 minutes. Add 1 cup of water, cover the skillet, and continue cooking for 10 minutes until the vegetables are wilted.

3. In a small bowl, dissolve the arrowroot powder in the remaining ½ cup of water, then add the arrowroot mixture to the vegetables and cook for 2 to 3 minutes. Stir constantly until the sauce thickens and becomes glossy. Add the sesame oil, vinegar, and honey, and then serve.

**Nutrition Facts:** Total calories 174, protein 35 g, carbs 34 g, fat 13 g,  saturated fat 3 g, fiber 8 g, salt 0.2 g.

# Paleo-style Cobb Salad

Another great dinner recipe that's easy to prepare and yet highly nutritious, this Paleo-approved Cobb salad recipe should accompany you on most nights when you don't feel like spending too much time in the kitchen for a great dinner meal.

**Yield:** 4 servings

**Ingredients:**

1 small size chicken breast, cooked

6 large romaine lettuce leaves, sliced

1 cup cherry tomatoes, halved

1 avocado, diced

4 hard-boiled eggs, quartered

8 pcs. turkey bacon, cooked, crumbled

ranch dressing, homemade

**Directions:**

1. Dice the chicken breast into ½-inch cubes.
2. On 4 plates, lay down the lettuce and then top with the chicken breast, tomatoes and avocado. Sprinkle bacon crumbles onto each of the 4

individual servings of salad and drizzle with ranch dressing.

3. Decorate by placing egg wedges on the outer rim of each plate and then serve.

**Nutrition Facts:** Total calories 115, protein 31 g, carbs 17 g, fat 4 g,  saturated fat 0 g, fiber 11 g, salt 0 g.

# Mango Chicken

We don't often think of fruits and meat as compatible ingredients in one dish but this just depends on how you work with the available ingredients. Here, we combined chicken and mango to show that common ingredients can be easily integrated with just a few culinary tricks.

**Yield:** 4 servings

**Ingredients:**

1 ¼ pound chicken breast, cut

¼ cup olive oil

1 large onion, chopped

1 red bell pepper, diced

2 garlic cloves, sliced

1 tbsp. fresh ginger, minced

1 tsp. curry powder

1 tsp. Celtic sea salt

1 tbsp. apple cider vinegar

1 cup water

½ cup coconut milk

1 mango, peeled, diced

**Directions:**

1. In a large pan, add olive oil over medium heat and sauté the onions for about 5 minutes, stirring occasionally. Add the red pepper, ginger, garlic, curry and salt, and cook for another 5 minutes. Continue adding the vinegar, water, coconut milk and mango to the pan and then bring the whole mixture to a boil then then reduce heat. Add the chicken pieces and allow to simmer for about 10 minutes until the chicken is cooked through.

2. Garnish with cilantro and serve.

**Nutrition Facts:** Total calories 176, protein 32 g, carbs 28 g, fat 8 g, saturated fat 1 g, fiber 7 g, salt 0.8 g.

# Rosemary-Apple Chicken

This is a great chicken roast recipe that you can prepare on family-dinner night. Roasting the chicken takes some time to make sure to prepare the ingredients beforehand in order to facilitate cooking and reduce the waiting time.

**Yield:** 6 servings

**Ingredients:**

1 whole chicken

¼ cup olive oil

¼ cup balsamic vinegar

1 tbsp. Celtic sea salt

4 apples, cored, sliced

4 sprigs rosemary

**Directions:**

1. Rinse the chicken, then pat dry with a paper towel and place on a baking dish. Drizzle with oil and vinegar, then sprinkle with salt. Arrange the apples around the chicken in the baking dish and place the sprigs of rosemary under the chicken.

2. Bake at 350°F for about 90 minutes until brown.

3. Serve.

**Nutrition Facts:** Total calories 143, <u>protein 75 g,</u> carbs 29 g, fat 10 g, saturated fat 3 g, fiber 6 g, salt 0.6 g.

# Fish Sticks

Who doesn't like fish sticks? Just make a great dip and this is already a perfect light dinner or a companion to a salad. Enjoy!

**Yield:** 4 servings

**Ingredients:**

    1 pound white fish

    2 eggs, whisked

    1 cup almond flour, blanched

    1 tsp. Celtic sea salt

    ¼ cup olive oil

    ¼ cup grapeseed oil

**Directions:**

1. Rinse the fish fillets in cold water and set on a plate. Cut them into sticks.

2. In one, place eggs and flour and salt in another. Dip the fish sticks in egg, then on to the flour and then onto a plate.

3. Mix the grapeseed oil and olive oil in a large skillet over medium high. Fry half of the fish sticks in the pan leaving enough room around

them so that they aren't crowded. Cook for a few minutes on each side until browned, then remove the fish sticks to a plate lined with a paper towel. Continue frying the remaining batch of fish sticks.

4. Serve with ketchup or homemade mayonnaise depending on your preference.

**Nutrition Facts:** Total calories 172, protein 35 g, carbs 26 g, fat 11 g, saturated fat 3 g, fiber 4 g, salt 0.5 g.

# Chicken Meatballs

We're used to meatballs made from other types of meat so it's time to expand your culinary repertoire by adding this chicken meatballs recipe to your arsenal. Remember; you can always use this to garnish other recipes like your favorite salad in order to create a perfect meal.

**Yield:** 4 servings

**Ingredients:**

1 zucchini, chopped

2 carrots, chopped

½ cup parsley, coarsely chopped

3 medium cloves garlic

¼ cup blanched almond flour

1 egg

1 pound chicken breasts, boneless, skinless

1 tsp. Celtic sea salt

½ tsp. ground pepper

¼ tsp. chili powder

**Directions:**

1. Preheat your oven to 350°F.

2. In a food processor, process the zucchini, carrots, parsley and garlic together, then add the almond flour, egg, and chicken. Continue pulsing with the salt, pepper and chili powder and process until thoroughly combined.

3. Form tablespoon-sized meatballs from the mixture and put into a plate lined with a baking sheet. Bake the meatballs for about 25 minutes. Serve.

**Nutrition Facts:** Total calories 164, protein 38 g, carbs 27 g, fat 10 g,  saturated fat 3 g, fiber 7 g, salt 0.7 g.

# Orange-and-Ginger Chicken

You can never have too many chicken recipes in your arsenal, particularly for dinner when picking the right meat that will cook quickly is very important after a long day at the office. In that view, here's an orange-and-ginger chicken recipe that you can rely on days when you need fruit and meat together on a plate.

**Yield:** 6 servings

**Ingredients:**

    1 whole chicken

    1 tsp. orange zest

    1 cup orange juice

    2 tbsp. agave nectar

    1 tbsp. ume plum vinegar

    2 tbsp. orange jam

    1 tbsp. ginger, fresh minced

    1 tbsp. garlic, finely minced

    1 tbsp. grapeseed oil or olive oil

    1 fresh orange, to garnish

**Directions:**

1. Place the chicken in a baking dish.
2. Combine the zest, juice, agave, vinegar, jam, ginger, garlic and grapeseed oil together in a medium bowl and pour over chicken. Marinate the chicken in the refrigerator for 3 hours.
3. Bake the chicken at 350°F for 60 minutes spooning sauce over chicken at 15 minute intervals. Turn off the oven and let the chicken sit in the oven for one half hour to set juices.
4. To serve, transfer the chicken to a platter and garnish with fresh orange slices.

**Nutrition Facts:** Total calories 161, <u>protein 44 g,</u> carbs 29 g, fat 12 g, saturated fat 1 g, fiber 5 g, salt 0.3 g.

# Example Of The 7-Day Paleo Meal Plan

So now we have the recipes; try this sample paleo meal plan to help you maximize your fitness potential, while having enough protein to promote and build lean muscle mass.

| Day | Breakfast | Afternoon | Dinner |
|-----|-----------|-----------|--------|
| 1 | Banana Paleo Shake | Tuna Steaks | Rosemary-Apple Chicken |
| 2 | Paleo Porridge | Baked Salmon | Chicken Meatballs |
| 3 | Apple-Carrot-Banana Bread | Shrimp and Spinach Salad | Paleo-Style Cobb Salad |
| 4 | Protein-Rich Paleo Pumpkin Pancakes | Meat Lover's Chili | Orange-and-Ginger Chicken |
| 5 | Poached Egg with Peace and Prosciutto Salsa | Chicken Salad | Asian Stir-Fry |
| 6 | Paleo Breakfast | The Ultimate | Fish Sticks |

|   | Casserole | Paleo Meatloaf | |
|---|---|---|---|
| 7 | Paleo Omelet | Paleo-Approved Jambalaya | Mango Chicken |

# Conclusion

If you are an everyday athlete, you can certainly benefit from a great diet that is rich in protein as well as a balance of nutrients. Protein is essential for muscle-building and as an athlete, you can never turn your back on that. In addition, you need a balanced diet to help fuel your workouts and your recovery.

That's where the Paleo diet becomes a perfect fit! The Caveman's diet is a great eating habit that takes advantage of readily available food sources to create a fulfilling and nourishing diet that can help you become a better "everyday athlete." Whether you're competing against yourself to beat a personal record or you're serious about scoring a podium finish at a local race, the Paleo diet is guaranteed to only make you better at what you do.

To kickstart your Paleo habit, you can refer to the 7-day Paleo plan here. Beyond that, you can regularly cook your own Paleo meals using the recipes outlined here. Embracing the Paleo takes some adjustment but if you keep at it, you should be able to see significant results in as little as 3 weeks.

Lastly, always be mindful of the ingredients you use. Fresh ingredients are not-negotiable. If you can wean your body from processed foods, that would lead to more dramatic results in the long-run.

Enjoy, and cheers to a healthy and long life as an everyday athlete fueled by the Paleo diet!

# Enjoy this book?

**Please leave a review below and let us know what you liked about this book by clicking on the Amazon image below.**

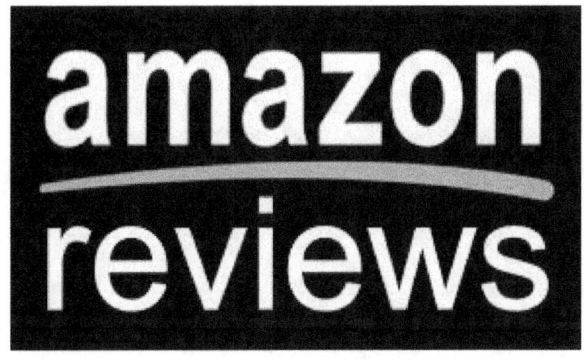

*and click on Digital Orders.*

*The above link directs to Amazon.com. Please change the .com to your own country extension.*